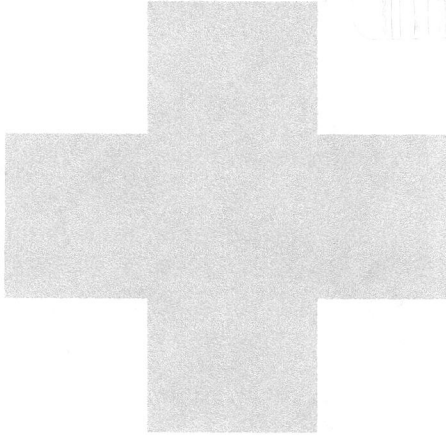

THE
HEALTHCARE
LITTLE BLACK BOOK

10 Secrets to a Better Healthcare Experience

Preethy Kaibara MD, Esq.

TPK

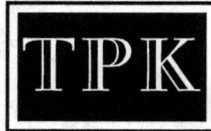

TPK LLC
3219 E. Camelback Rd. #789
Phoenix, AZ 85018

ISBNs:
Paperback 978-0-9861442-0-2
Digital 978-0-9861442-1-9

For my three little birds.

FOREWORD

First disclosure: This is a simple book.

Second disclosure: The secrets in these pages exist elsewhere, but they're scattered through books, journals, websites, health blogs, articles, social media … you get the picture. Is it anything and everything you need to know about the healthcare system? Of course not. But, here—in short form and in one place—are critical steps to help you achieve more quality and value from your healthcare.

Each chapter covers a single "secret" and ends with a "Resource Box" that lists websites to help further explore the topic. Some chapters also contain a worksheet to apply that topic practically to your own circumstances. Please remember, this book intends to guide you through, but never to substitute for, your healthcare experiences.

As a family doctor and healthcare lawyer, I have seen great successes and big disappointments from our healthcare system. As there are many books on the disappointments, I sincerely hope this book contributes to your successes.

To you in health,
Preethy Kaibara M.D., Esq.

CONTENTS

CHAPTER 1
Make a Health Record

Everything should be made as simple as possible, but not simpler.
Albert Einstein

Perhaps you can recall a time when you were a patient and had to answer the same questions repeatedly. You might have wondered whether anyone actually read your chart. Some repetition is necessary to make sure you are not deathly allergic to a medicine or to confirm which eye needs to be operated on.

However, I can recall too many instances when I read "no past medical history" on a patient's chart, only to find a maze of surgical scars on the patient's body during my examination.

When you bring in a summary of your health history when you receive care, it creates an opportunity to reduce both errors like this and needless repetition. This chapter guides you through the process of compiling your health history. Once you've completed the worksheet at the end of this chapter, congratulations! You are the proud owner of a **Personal Health Record** (**PHR** for short).

You may have heard the term **Electronic Health Record (EHR)**. These are the electronic records kept by hospitals and medical offices. The problem with EHRs is that different offices, hospitals, labs, and radiology facilities have a part of your health history—but not the whole thing. Really, the only person who is constantly part of your healthcare is you. You are the very best person to create the most complete medical record. If your health is complex, you travel a lot, or you're planning to move, a PHR will be worth its weight in gold. Here are some steps to make your own PHR:

1. Write down what you already know. You need the highlights, not every detail of your past health (your **Past Medical History**). The details can stay in your doctors' or hospitals' records. For example, you don't need to include the two stitches in your pinky after that unfortunate incident with a tuna can. You should include serious childhood illnesses, any condition where you had to stay overnight in the hospital for care (**admitted**), and any condition that requires regular or even semi-regular medication. List all surgical procedures you've had and if there were any complications. Include suspicious mole removals, as well as complex dental and plastic surgeries.

You may not remember your past immunizations, but going forward (and with all young children and their PHRs), keep track of the date, type of immunization, and manufacturer of the immunization. This is helpful because the recommended immunization schedule changes and expands with some regularity. New vaccines replace older ones because they provide a longer immunity. In other instances, completely new vaccines appear. For example, the chicken pox is a current, routine childhood vaccine that was not around for most adults who are now over 40 years of age.

Your medication list should include all current medications, vitamins, and any over-the-counter supplements you take (because many can interact with prescription medications). Write down the **dose** (not the number of pills) and the number of times you take that dose a day.

To figure out your dose, look on the pill bottle for the strength of the pills and multiply that by the number of pills you take at one time. The number of pills is not as useful because most pills come in multiple strengths. If you took a medication and had a reaction to it, list it in your allergies section along with the type of reaction (rash, difficulty breathing, etc.). Some allergies extend to other classes of drugs you could be prescribed that would result in a similar reaction. Also, list any serious food or environmental allergies.

You don't need to include medications you have taken in the past and discontinued without any problems, such as antibiotics. An exception to this general rule is if you have a chronic medical condition and you have tried a number of different kinds of medications. You don't want to have to retry the same class of drugs again. High blood pressure, migraine headaches, Parkinson's disease, and chronic pain are all examples of chronic conditions where there's often a lot of trial and error with drugs before you find one that works. For chronic pain, knowing what medications have not worked will help your healthcare team select the right class of pain medications and reduce the risk of pain medication addiction.

Test results can be more difficult to sort out, but knowing key results can help you avoid having to repeat tests. If a repeat test is necessary, knowing your earlier results can also help your providers compare and interpret your current results. This can be true for:

- **Blood test results**

- "Scope" tests where your insides are viewed with a long tube attached to a camera—e.g., colonoscopies (colon), **gastroscopies** (stomach), and **bronchoscopies** (lungs)

- **Radiographs (X-Rays,** which are pictures of your bones and tissues, created by radiation beams)

- **Computerized Tomography Scan** (**CT scan,** which is a second generation X-ray with more detail of your body)

- **Magnetic Resonance Image** (**MRI,** which is a detailed picture of the soft tissues, created without radiation)

- **Electrocardiograms** (**ECG or EKG,** which is an electrical tracing of your heart) and other cardiac tests (e.g., stress testing, cardiac angiograms, and thallium testing)

Request a copy of test results from the location where you did the test. Sometimes they can give you your results on a compact disc or DVD. Going forward, ask the testing center to send you a copy of the results right when you have a test.

Next on your PHR, include diseases that run in your family (your **Family History**). Alternatively, if you do not know what diseases (e.g., you are adopted or other circumstances), include this fact because this is just as important. Some important categories of hereditary diseases are cancers, heart disease, sudden unexplained death, kidney problems, diabetes, immunologic disorders, and neurologic diseases. Include family death or illness under age 65.

Some **Social History** should also be in your PHR. This includes use or past use of alcohol, tobacco, and recreational and prescription drugs (those not prescribed to you), as well as your history of sexually transmitted diseases. This is personal stuff, but it can significantly change what treatments are best or should be avoided when you need healthcare. Remember, too, that healthcare professionals have a legal and ethical duty to keep your health information confidential. Tell the doctor your social history if you would prefer not to have it in writing.

2. Discuss your PHR. Once you have started your PHR, it's helpful to run it past a doctor to see where you should include more information. You could also review your medication list with your pharmacist. These steps allow you to fine-tune your request for medical records, which is the next step. This can save you copying costs, time sifting through paperwork, and ultimately your sanity. A request for "My last blood count in December 2010" or "My chest X-ray report dated May 17, 2011" is much easier to manage than asking for "All of my records in 2010 and 2011." Your doctor may even have some of these results on file to share with you.

In the case of chronic conditions (such as diabetes, heart disease, or lung disease), ask the doctor what tests results are important for you to track. For example, if you have heart disease, your most recent **cholesterol** (a type of fat found in your blood), blood pressure value, and heart tracing (**EKG**) are important parts of your PHR because regular testing, with proper management of abnormalities, reduces your risk of complications.

A copy of your results can be incredibly valuable in emergencies too. Having your most recent EKG gives the emergency room a baseline, which can make interpreting your emergency room EKG more accurate and timely. When you are having chest pain, changes in your EKG tracing are critical to deciding whether or not you are having a heart attack. What good is that EKG from just last month if it's in your doctor's office and no one can access it at two in the morning?

Similarly, if you are diabetic, you should have annual eye exams to reduce the risk of blindness from diabetes. Keeping track of the results yourself helps double-check that you have that yearly exam and helps you follow the progress of your diabetes.

3. Get a copy of the records you need to fill in the gaps. Access to your medical records is your legal right, but getting them can be a frustrating process. You may have to sign a permission form and pay a copying fee. (It has to be reasonable by law.) As discussed earlier, try to request records right at the time of service whenever possible because it is the simplest way for you to get a copy.

Start by requesting records from the office of your admitting doctor or the surgeon who looked after you. Ask for the final record of your stay, called the **discharge summary.** A discharge summary includes the highlights of your admission and/or surgery and may be all you need.

If you still need more records, you may need to contact your hospital's **medical records department.** Because these records are frequently housed somewhere inconvenient such as in a basement room, it's best to call ahead and find out what you need to do to obtain your records. Expect that you'll be asked to fill out paperwork and that you may need to wait several days before they are ready for pick-up.

Generally, hospital records include many details that are not necessary for your PHR. Again, try to request specific records from specific dates and discharge summaries to minimize your time sorting through a pile of paper. If this seems too difficult, many hospitals now have an advocate office whose job it is to help answer patient questions. Finally, ask your doctor if you need more help getting the records you need.

4. Organize your PHR. The simplest and most private PHR option is just to write your health information down on a piece of paper (like the Worksheet included here). The disadvantage of the paper approach is that you have to keep making new ones and you have to carry it with you for it to be useful. Another option is to create a document on your computer and easily edit it as necessary. You then can save the information on a memory device (such as a flash drive) and carry it with you. Either way, consider keeping a copy of your PHR in your car and, ideally, in your wallet or purse.

An alternate approach is to create an online PHR, which is accessible at any time on the Internet and can be printed when necessary.

It's initially more tedious than writing out your history, but it gets easier once you have set it up and you only have to make updates.

The key advantage is that online PHRs have greater potential uses. For example, many online PHRs have a feature to authorize health-care providers to look at your PHR online when you are ill. Some sites enable you to attach devices to your computer, like blood-pressure and blood-sugar machines, and automatically upload the results to your records. This allows you to track your progress and share the information with your doctor without a lot of manual work.

Some people have privacy concerns about online PHRs. This is completely valid as there is no such thing as foolproof Internet security. In this chapter's Resource Box, I've included some free versions of PHRs that have adopted high levels of online security. Many private PHR companies offer added benefits (e.g., bracelets, storage of wills and other documents, live operator help, etc.). Search for these on the Internet if you find them of interest.

WORKSHEET

My Personal Health Record

Name/Date of Birth: _____

Medications (include vitamins and supplements):

Name	Dose Amount	Times a Day	Notes

I am allergic to and my reaction is (drugs, foods, and environmental):

_____

Past Medical History (include number of years for each condition, vaccinations, and every hospital admission):

_____
_____
_____
_____

Past Surgical History (include date and any complications**):**

_____

_____

_____

Test Results (EKGs, X-rays, blood tests, etc.**):** _____

_____

_____

Family History (include how you are related to them**):**

People in my family have died before age 65 from:

_____

Many family members have had these diseases:

_____

Social History:

I drink/used to drink _____ alcoholic drinks per week.

I smoke/used to smoke _____ packs/week for _____ years.

I use /have used the following street drugs or prescriptions not pre-scribed to me: _____

_____.

I have had the following sexually transmitted diseases: _____

_____.

RESOURCE BOX
Personal Health Records

medicalert.org—Provides jewelry and devices with important medical information imprinted on them in case you are unable to speak for yourself (e.g., a wristband or necklace).

healthvault.com—An always-expanding PHR site. It includes mobile phone apps for health and fitness, can communicate with pharmacies, and allows uploading of data from certain medical devices (e.g., blood-glucose and blood-pressure devices).

patientfusion.com—A free PHR that has the potential to integrate your doctors' records, and some insurance plan records, into your PHR.

CHAPTER 2
Use the Internet

Be careful about reading health books. You may die of a misprint.
Mark Twain

The beauty of the Internet is how much information you have access to in the privacy of your own home. The problem with the Internet is also how much information you have access to in the privacy of your own home. With all that access comes the risk of information overload and misinformation.

For example, search "headaches" and you'll get more than twenty million results. Talk about information overload. This can easily lead to **hypochondria**—diagnosing yourself with a terrible and rare disease to explain your common symptoms. With few Internet police officers, websites with hidden sales agendas and wrong information are mixed among the sites with good information. This chapter lays out how best to avoid these pitfalls and use the Internet to your advantage.

1. Start with health search engines. This will reduce your hits from millions of matching results on a general search engine to thousands, save you time, and improve the quality of information to choose from. The Resource Box at the end of this chapter lists some reliable websites.

2. Look beyond the website name. A powerful name does not always translate to being the best site. For example, arthritis.com sounds like *the* website for arthritis. However, a company that sells arthritis drugs created it. This does not mean the information is bad, but it is limited. For example, the website will probably not be comprehensive about competitor drugs or non-drug alternatives to treatment.

On the other hand, websites with ".gov" at the end are often better information sources. These are government agency websites, which can be a useful and objective place to start research on both disease and the healthcare system. Similarly, ".org" sites can indicate a non-profit organization that will present unbiased information. However, there is little regulation of who can use ".org," so keep reading for further ways to evaluate these websites.

3. Examine the layout of the website. Is it organized and logical? When was it last updated (usually at the bottom right or left corner of the home screen)? Most good sources will tell you when the information was last updated, and it should be recent. Some websites that offer information on absolutely everything present health information in a disorganized way, with too many links and paid advertising for ideal health research.

4. Credentials are good, but they are not everything. Good sites use many different experts. The lone-doctor site may be more opinion than fact. Is the advice one-sided or designed to tell you that he, or she, is the only one in the whole world who knows what to do and can sell you the products to do it? Such sites prey on people's vulnerability, especially people suffering from a complex problem or who have few treatment options. Many emotional patient testimonials can be a clue that you've come across one of these websites.

5. Read the fine print. Check the "About Us" tab on the site to review whose advice you're reading. Look at the advisors and writers. Are they mainly medical professionals? Another good sign is the "URAC Accredited Health Website"© or "HonCode"© (Health on the Net Foundation). These designations mean that (excluding government websites) the website adheres to safe consumer health information practices.

6. Search often. Searching is like working on a research project. New devices and medications come on the market all the time and slowly trickle down to healthcare providers. You may stumble upon options to treat your condition that are unknown to your healthcare provider. For example, your doctor may be aware of the medications to treat migraines, but may not know about a new electric headband device that has similar effects on migraines as many medications. You can bring innovative treatments to the table now more than ever.

7. Second-opinion yourself. Find at least two separate sources that support a conclusion or diagnosis that you have made. This is a good check and balance of the reliability of the information.

8. Make a plan. How would you rate the seriousness of your problem? For example, if you are having bloody stools, this is a 10/10 on the seriousness scale, and you should see a healthcare provider as soon as possible. Some other important symptoms not to ignore are unexplained weight loss or gain, bleeding, chest pain, and neurologic symptoms. If nothing is outright concerning at this time, is there something you learned from your Internet research that would allow you to try an at-home method to help your problem? If so, you might try that method for a week and make note of any differences. If the problem continues or changes, see a healthcare professional.

RESOURCE BOX
Examples of Websites with Reliable Health Information

medlineplus.gov—National Institute of Health site where you can search for information by disease, sex, and age.

familydoctor.org—An American Academy of Family Physicians searchable website with health information for all ages.

webmd.com—Information on symptoms, diseases, and lifestyle modifications.

uptodate.com—Use the "Patients and Caregivers" section to find recent research on medical topics.

kidshealth.org—A children's health website that is searchable by parents, children, and teens.

nichd.nih.gov—Use the "Parents, Patients, and Caregivers" link to access this National Institute of Health website and explore children's health and development topics.

Many large hospitals (e.g., Mayo Clinic, Cleveland Clinic) have information about health topics on their websites, as do many specialty organizations (e.g., American Cancer Society, American Diabetes Association, American Heart Association).

CHAPTER 3
Heal Yourself

Natural forces within us are the true healers of disease.

Hippocrates

Somewhere between going to the emergency room (ER) for a splinter and removing your own appendix is a whole bunch of methods for self-care that you are most likely capable of. There's nothing sexy in this chapter; the issues discussed below are very common reasons for visits to the doctor and the emergency room. If you are generally healthy (not very young, very old, or suffering from a serious or chronic condition), then consider the suggestions discussed here.

1. Trust your gut. The starting point is that if something just feels off to you, ignore this chapter and seek medical attention. Let your instincts be your guide. There are two particular conditions where time equals health. These are heart attacks and brain strokes, where time is of the essence. If you get emergency treatment during the **golden hour**—the first hour after an attack occurs—you have a better chance of avoiding permanent and irreversible damage (such as paralysis or irreversible heart damage).

2. Use antibiotics sparingly. The odds are that a virus caused your runny nose, aches, chills, sore throat, and cough. Many studies prove this. Viruses do not get better with antibiotics. Viruses get better over time. Even green mucous is not a sure sign that your illness is bacterial, because some kinds of fighter blood cells release greenish-colored enzymes to fight viruses.

For example, sinus pain and drainage that occur fewer than ten days are, 90 percent of the time, related to a viral problem, and yet nearly 20 percent of US antibiotic prescriptions are for sinus infections. Fluids, pain relief, and saline nasal sprays or irrigation are better treatment choices.

Using antibiotics for just-in-case situations has invisible negative consequences. Our bodies have important natural bacteria all over to protect us from illness. Antibiotics inadvertently kill some of these bacteria because there is no way for the drug to tell the good guys from the bad guys (think of going after a target with a bomb rather than a sniper). Many women feel this loss of protection because whenever they take antibiotics, they get a yeast infection. This happens because good bacteria found in the genital tract died from the antibiotic taken for some other reason (e.g., for an ear infection).

In addition, taking antibiotics when you don't need them reduces their effectiveness for when you really do. Bacteria smartly learn how to neutralize the effect of an antibiotic with each exposure. This is **antibiotic resistance**, which creates what the media like to call "superbugs." Superbugs are bacteria that are resistant to antibiotics, and the worst of the bunch are the "flesh-eating bacteria" you sometimes hear about. These are bacteria with few or *no* antibiotics available to treat them.

Many doctors will admit to feeling pressure to write prescriptions for antibiotics. I've made some patients unhappy when I've suggested that antibiotics were not necessary. I can understand the frustration. They don't feel well, they took time off work, and they probably waited too long to see a doctor. It becomes easy to assume that every patient expects a prescription. In contrast, I've had patients complain that they get handed a prescription within three minutes of sitting down to discuss their problem with a doctor. By telling the doctor up front that you do not necessarily want antibiotics but you do want an opinion, you clear the air on this issue and together make the best decision on whether or not you should take antibiotics.

The bottom line is that when you are ill, fluids, pain relievers, rest, and patience for forty-eight hours will get you over the hump 90 percent of the time. Patience is probably the biggest challenge, since we all lead busy lives.

If you improve with this regimen, or at least are no worse, consider holding off on a doctor visit. If you absolutely need an office visit because of work, travel, kids, or other reasons, discuss a **safe script** with your doctor. This is a prescription that you will try not to fill unless your symptoms worsen or change. Research shows that safe scripts are actually filled by patients less than 50 percent of the time.

3. Have an ache? Try RICE for a week. The acronym RICE stands for **R**est (stop doing whatever makes you say, "It hurts when I do this"), **I**ce (an ice pack covered with a towel or a frozen veggie package works great), **C**ompression (e.g.,a splint or elastic wrap), and **E**levation (get the hurting part up on a pillow or chair every chance you get). If you are able to bear weight on an ankle or foot, it's less likely broken than sprained. If the body part gets better every day, it's also less likely broken than sprained. Use pain relief medications such as ibuprofen as directed on the bottle (unless you have a condition prohibiting the use of this class of medication, like kidney disease or a medication allergy). All of these things reduce inflammation and swelling, which are the sources of the pain. If you are getting worse, not better, or if the pain persists after a week, consult a doctor.

4. Treat nutrition as medicine. Food is more than fuel for the body. It's your daily medicine. Nutritional advice today has gone slightly wacky because it's a multi-million dollar business. We're bombarded with news about the latest superfood, antioxidant, or miracle supplement. Today red wine is a health savior; tomorrow it's deadly. I know of a person who once ate so much canned tuna (she wanted to increase her fish oil consumption), she managed to give herself mercury poisoning. Her problem became clear when she began losing handfuls of hair.

Problems like hers occur because nutrition is complex, and restrictive diets can lead to deficiencies or build-ups of trace minerals and vitamins. Many vitamins are water-soluble, so taking a vitamin supplement in addition to eating means your body uses what it needs and turns the rest into expensive pee. Other nutrients are fat soluble, meaning excess will build up in your fat stores and potentially interfere with normal cell function and repair.

Some nutrition experts argue that with all of the nutrient-fortified food and drinks out there, most people end up with much more than the **recommended daily allowance (RDA)** of many nutrients. We are just beginning to explore what the consequences of this will be. For example, vitamin E was once all the rage to help prevent dementia. However, most research has found that vitamin E supplements do not improve health and actually increase the risk of death overall. Bottom line, there is no wonder food or supplement that will cure all that ails you or prevent all disease. Stay sane and ignore the hype.

In contrast, many people eat a lot of food with very little nutritional value. It's not a newsflash that many Americans are obese. The more we obsess about losing weight, the less success we seem to have.

Whatever the cause of nationally poor nutrition, the result has been excess weight for many people. For many Americans, this can result in **Type 2 (or non-insulin dependent) diabetes** and high blood pressure. Research has shown that even as little as a 7-percent body weight loss can reverse Type 2 diabetes. That means that an overweight person with Type 2 diabetes who weighs two hundred pounds can lose fourteen pounds and stand a chance of curing their diabetes. Similarly, lowering your salt intake can lower your blood pressure up to ten points and may allow you to stay off blood pressure pills. Nearly all processed food has salt in it—even the sweet kind!

So prescribe yourself the good nutrition. As with medications, generics are a great starting point. In the case of food, generics are whole foods. Eat the apple, not the apple bar fortified with vitamins and minerals. Where whole foods are not possible, find packaged foods with fewer than five items on the ingredients list. The first two cannot be sodium, sugar, fructose, glucose, high fructose corn syrup, or dextrose.

The second aspect of a prescription is quantity. Less is more. Typical restaurant portions are much larger than the ideal portion. Use smaller dinner plates, drink water before eating, and pack half of your meal in a to-go box. These are just a few strategies to avoid taking in too many calories.

5. Exercise is not just for weight loss. Incredibly, even without a pound of weight loss, exercise alone can reduce your blood pressure, lower high cholesterol, and stabilize your blood sugar. Women who do weight-bearing exercises reduce their chances of hip and other fractures as they age. Elderly people who exercise are less likely to acquire dementia. Safe exercise is simply a no-brainer to improving your health.

Unfortunately, our modern lifestyle has many of us plunked down at computers during the day and driving nearly everywhere. You have to find time to exercise. Start with ten minutes a day and work up to thirty minutes. You don't need a pricey gym membership to exercise. Stairs and the outdoors are free, or find a home workout on the Internet. You should move every day.

6. There's an app for that. If measuring things helps you stay on course, consider a fitness-tracker device (watches or bands) and the health apps in your smart phone's applications store. Search the store for terms like "medical apps" and "medical tools," or search your specific disease. New applications appear regularly, so ideally search a few times a year. Read the customer reviews of the app to see if others have found it useful, especially if you have to pay for it. Sometimes the premium version of the app costs a few dollars. Try the free version and if you are finding it useful, it may be worth it.

7. Treat sleep as medicine. Studies on the importance of sleep are everywhere. Chronic pain, excess weight, and accidents are just a few examples of problems that improve with enough sleep. Your cells need time to rest and repair, and the best time for that is during sleep.

8. DIY medicine. A new patient experience in medicine is something I call **DIY** medicine (**do-it-yourself** medicine). For example, you can order a test online, go to a lab to have it done, and receive the results. On the upside, this is empowering, convenient, and often cheaper than traditional healthcare. Tracking ovulation and allergy testing are just a couple of DIY tests available that are less expensive than the traditional healthcare version.

Nevertheless, testing is a dangerous mistress. You may be falsely reassured that you do not have the condition (a **false negative**) or falsely alarmed that you do have the condition (a **false positive**). This is not a big problem if you are testing for allergies, but other conditions may have bigger consequences if incorrectly self-diagnosed. For example, there are DIY tests for a **urinary tract infection** (**UTI**). In a healthy person with a history of UTI, this can be a simple way to confirm what you know. However, the same symptoms could signal kidney disease or a sexually transmitted disease that needs more in-depth treatment. So approach DIY testing carefully and try not to overuse it. Mix it up with in-person care, particularly if your symptom is a serious one, persists, or has changed.

In addition to false positives and negatives, **incidental findings** are another drawback to consider before you test yourself. An incidental finding is something noted on a test that is not technically normal, but is unrelated to why the test was done. For example, a total body CT is a DIY test marketed as a way to know what diseases are hiding in your body. Putting aside that healthcare professionals rarely order this test and the large amount of radiation to the body (several dozen X-rays), this test often spots tiny incidental findings. The kidney, for example, can have serious or harmless (**benign**) tumors. If you had benign tumors but you didn't know they existed, you could happily coexist with them. But once a test turned up those irregularities, you'd need further tests before the healthcare system could tell you that you had nothing to worry about.

Another DIY example is chatting with an online doctor to ask a medical question. This is certainly a convenient way to talk to a doctor for simple conditions, and it could be a useful way to get a second opinion from a specialist expert. However, an online chat is a brief, virtual encounter. Be mindful of whether the particular problem you have would be better suited to an in-person visit.

Many private companies out there offer an ever-expanding list of DIY services. Just search the Internet for things like "order lab tests online" or "see a doctor online." Review chapter 2 to decide whether the website looks trustworthy.

Genetic testing is another DIY service. The test results can give you information on diseases you have or are at risk for. In some cases, you have some control over the disease, such as diabetes or heart disease.

In 2013, genetic testing entered the popular media spotlight when Angelina Jolie elected to have both of her breasts removed (a **bilateral mastectomy**) because she found she had a gene that increased her risk of breast cancer.

On the other hand, you could discover you have a gene for a disease for which you cannot do anything to reduce risk. Some people would like to know about the risk ahead of time, while others would not. Consider the impact of genetic testing results on close relatives; your children and siblings may not want to know their risk of disease they cannot do anything to prevent. Aside from personal beliefs, life insurance and health insurance companies require you to disclose what you know about your health, and a known genetic risk could affect your premiums and insurance choices.

The decision to do genetic testing is thus personal and complex. What exactly does an increased risk mean for the gene you have? How far are you willing to go to reduce your risk? Should you share the results with other family members? The ideal way to explore these types of questions is with a **genetic counselor** before you do the test. The counselor will help you decide what tests to consider and the possible consequences, and can help you interpret the results. DIY genetic testing does not provide genetic counseling, so look at the websites in this chapter's Resource Box to help you decide if it's a good option for you.

RESOURCE BOX

ghr.nlm.nih.gov—The National Institute of Health site, which gives unbiased information on genetic conditions and information about screening and counseling.

nsgc.org—The National Society of Genetic Counselors website, where you can learn more about genetic counseling and find a genetic counselor in your area.

CHAPTER 4
Master Your Medications

It is easy to get a thousand prescriptions but hard to get one single remedy.
Chinese Proverb

Medications are the workhorse of modern medicine. The list of medications keeps growing, but so do the costs and complications. This chapter discusses how to make the most of your medications while reducing costs and potential complications.

1. Know your non-drug options. There are many conditions for which a lifestyle change is a better treatment than medication. Recall from chapter 3 that a person with Type 2 diabetes may avoid diabetic medication by losing just 7 percent of his body weight. High cholesterol (**hypercholesterolemia**) and high blood pressure (**hypertension**) are other diseases for which exercise and diet can make a big difference. Research your options on the Internet and then talk to a doctor. There may be more options than you think (search the medical term for this, which is **lifestyle modifications**). For example, we commonly understand that lowering fat in your diet will reduce cholesterol, but so does increasing soluble fiber. Work with your doctor to track the effects of your lifestyle modifications. Generally, six months is a reasonable amount of time to see whether treatment without medications is realistic.

2. If medications are your only option, take them. There are many conditions where you might not feel that bad if you forget to take your medications, but you may suffer silent damage. For example, patients with hypertension often dislike how blood pressure medications initially make them feel. This discomfort is common while the body is adjusting to a lower blood pressure. But the consequence of high blood pressure is painless (and often irreversible) damage to the heart, kidneys, brain, and eyes, or a stroke or a heart attack.

3. Get to know your pharmacist. Your pharmacist will educate you on what food and drug interactions to watch for, and possible side effects of your medication. Use one pharmacy as much as possible to avoid drug interactions and to get important safety information. A good pharmacist will help you select simpler or cheaper options and even contact your doctor to request the change.

4. Look for ways to make taking your medication easier. Not taking your medication at all or incorrectly is **non-compliance** in medical lingo. I only take one medication a day, and I am guilty of bouts of non-compliance. If your doctor believes you are taking your medication correctly (but you are not), then he or she will think the medication is not working and will change your medication or add a new one. This means more visits to the doctor and the risk of new side effects in addition to added costs. If the side effects are the reason behind your noncompliance, tell your doctor. There are usually other options. For example, some men are non-compliant with blood pressure medicines because they interfere with erections. However, the doctor could change the blood pressure medicine to one less likely to cause this side effect.

The more often you need to take a medication, the more likely it is that you will be noncompliant. So always ask for the simplest medication regime possible. The ideal is once a day. Sometimes, there is no choice but to take a drug three or four times a day. If you have trouble remembering if you took the medication, ask the pharmacist to put the medication in a weekly blister pack (they may charge for this). Alternatively, buy a refillable pillbox with the days of the week separated into different containers to help keep track of your medications. If you have to take your medication when you are away from home, try setting a cell phone alarm as a reminder. Find other reminder options in the Resource Box at the end of this chapter.

Another common pitfall is to run out of medication and not have the time or money for another appointment to get a refill. Try to avoid running out by asking for a ninety-day prescription if possible and/or request as many refills as the doctor can reasonably prescribe. Many pharmacies offer phone and automatic refills and will call you when it is time to pick up your medicine. There are even mail-order services and delivery options. Check with your pharmacy to explore your choices.

5. Generic medications could save you money. More than half of the drugs used by Americans are non-name-brand products (**generic medications**). The Food and Drug Administration (**FDA**) monitors generic medications to confirm that they work to the same effect as the corresponding name-brand medication. Most studies have shown that generics also have similar side-effect rates as name brands.

All major pharmacies offer monthly supplies of generic drugs for four dollars (and ten dollars for a ninety-day supply). Quite annoyingly, each pharmacy has a different four-dollar drug list and some require that you sign up for a membership (usually less than twenty dollars per year) to access cheaper drugs. Most of this information is available on the pharmacy's website or by phone. If you have insurance, most pharmacies will charge you the standard insured drug price, even if the medication is on their four-dollar list. To be charged four dollars, you may need to ask the pharmacist not to run the charge through your insurance. The drawback is that you will lose the credit of the medication cost toward your insurance deductible. This is still probably the better cost option, but think this through based on your health needs (see chapter 10 for more on deductibles).

6. Discuss whether getting a medication sample is your best choice. Getting samples of medications is useful because you are able to try the medication at no cost and see if it works and if the side effects are reasonable. Samples are newer, name-brand medications protected by patent laws. They tend to be more expensive in order to recover the research costs that went into creating the new drug. It is worth discussing whether a new drug is the best choice for you or whether using the generic version would be better.

For example, metformin is the decades-old, affordable and well-studied generic drug to treat diabetes that we know is effective and safe in most people. There are many newer diabetes medications that are available by sample initially and then at a higher cost than metformin. If you are concerned about your ability to afford a sample drug long-term, (e.g., maybe you are leaving your job and losing your health insurance), ask about your generic options and decide with your doctor on the best choice.

7. If generic medications are not ideal, discuss the name-brand medication costs with your insurance plan. Some patients find that the name-brand drug works better than the generic. In addition, there are some conditions where for which the generic drug and the name brand are the same price. Insurance companies generally divide medications into pricing tiers based on how effective and safe they have categorized the medication. Generally, the cheapest tier is generics, and the most expensive tier is newer name-brand medications. Contact your insurance to learn what tier your drug is in and whether you can appeal what tier your prescribed drug falls into (usually this is a form you fill out with your doctor).

8. Do you try an online international pharmacy? Online international pharmacies sell drugs at lower cost than the same drug sold in the United States. Cholesterol medication is an example of a drug class that costs about 85 percent less if ordered online. Most of these medications come from India and China. Even Canadian online pharmacies often just import the medications they advertise from India or China. The risk is that the medication may be manufactured poorly (e.g., not pure) and harmful to you, or it may not even be the drug you ordered. Drugs sold from US sources must follow federal FDA regulations, whereas internationally sold drugs do not. However, India in particular follows the World Health Organization's and other high standards of manufacturing. There is potential for the online pharmacy option to work for you, but be aware of these risks.

9. Is research an option? In a clinical research study, you will get the drug free (see chapter 10 for a more in-depth discussion about clinical research trials).

10. If all else fails, go to the source. Most pharmaceutical companies have **Patient Assistance Programs** that offer drugs at reduced costs (requiring some forms filled out by you and your doctor). The Resource Box here lists websites where you can learn more and access the correct forms.

RESOURCE BOX

Drug Cost Research

bestbuydrugs.org—*Consumer Reports* website that lists comparable drugs and which are safest and most cost-effective. This site is a great starting point if you're looking for a cheaper or more effective alternative.

goodrx.com—Website and app that allows you to search for the best price and gives you coupons to use at the pharmacy to reduce costs.

rxoutreach.org—A nonprofit program to provide mail-order drugs at a more affordable price.

Tracking Medications

mediguard.org—A free database to enter your medications, track safety information (like interactions) and research drugs.

medisafe.com—Website and app to keep track of your medications that sends reminders to take them. It will also notify a third party if a medication dose is missed (great for caregivers or those with aging parents).

There are many mobile phone apps to track medications (for example **My Medications app**, free from the American Medical Association). Search "medications" in your phone's app-purchasing store for choices. Many apps can be set to remind other people, like caregivers and family members. Some apps will remind you when you are close to needing a refill and some will link you to your pharmacy.

Drug Company Cost Assistance

rxassist.org—A searchable database of what assistance program to apply to for a particular name-brand drug.

needymeds.org—Provides contact information for patient-assistance programs, as well as a variety of other information to help you reduce your drug costs.

CHAPTER 5
Choose and Use Doctors

Never go to a doctor whose office plants have died.
Erma Bombeck

It's quite possible that you've met with at least one doctor that you still despise. I apologize on behalf of the medical profession. However, I believe there is a great doctor out there for each person. This chapter offers suggestions on how to find the right fit for you.

It's common for people to see a few specialists, with each of them responsible for a different condition. An endocrinologist might help with your diabetes but doesn't tie that into your blood pressure management, because that's not what they treat. A cardiologist can treat your blood pressure but be less helpful with the depression you've had since your heart attack. The problem with this piecemeal approach is that no one really knows all of you and is able to help streamline your care, reduce costs, and avoid errors. This is **fragmented healthcare.**

A primary care physician (also called a **family doctor** or **family physician**) works with you to avoid fragmented healthcare. The right doctor for you will address your big-picture health and coordinate care among your specialists. Here are some suggestions on how to choose a primary care doctor and use them to further your healthcare goals (a discussion of specialty care follows this section).

1. How does primary care work with insurance? Most of us want our insurance company to pay for our doctor visits without having extra costs. This requires an **in-network** primary care physician, who must charge the insurance company a specific amount and not ask you to pay extra. Every insurance plan will give you a list of in-network primary care doctors in your area. If you see an out-of-network physician, you may have to pay the difference between what insurance would pay an in-network physician and the physician's actual bill. There may be times when you feel the extra payment is worth it, but it's important to be aware that staying in-network is your most cost-effective option.

2. Are you better suited to a non-traditional practice? If you do not have insurance, you can still have a primary care doctor. In fact, having one can help control your healthcare costs.

Urgent care (care in a facility that treats routine and some emergency conditions) and **emergency room (ER)** care (treatment in a hospital emergency department) are your only options without a primary care doctor. These are much more expensive ways to deal with everyday healthcare. Chapter 10 includes low-cost and no-cost ways to have primary care. Below are two novel styles of primary care available as well.

Direct primary care practices deliver primary care by a monthly membership fee rather than through insurance premiums. The monthly fee includes a certain amount of healthcare each month (e.g., two or three visits or phone calls) and applies whether or not you go to the doctor that month.

Another option is **concierge medicine,** where doctors or nurse practitioners are available around the clock for visits or phone calls and may do house calls. Many concierge services do not accept insurance and rather charge an annual fee and/or a per-visit fee. If you have a chronic disease or have difficulty getting to a doctor, this could be a helpful option.

The Resource Box at the end of this chapter outlines how to find the above services in your area. Keep in mind these are non-insurance options, which means you still need to think about insurance to cover medications, hospital, and specialist costs.

3. Review the State Licensing Board Information. The board governs every practicing professional of each type in the state. Each board has a public website where you can look up the name of the professional you are interested in and find out if there have been any problems associated with that license.

Find medical doctors (**MD**) and physician assistants (**PA**) on the website for the state's Board of Medicine. Osteopaths (**DO**) are either in a separate Board of Osteopathy or together with the MDs and PAs. Nurse practitioners (**NP**) are located on your state's Board of Nursing website. To find your local boards, just search your state, the word "board," and the type of healthcare professional. There is an option located on the home page to search professionals by name.

MDs and DOs have studied medicine and are licensed to prescribe medications. They went to medical school, then completed clinical training in a hospital (a **residency**), and maybe underwent more specialized training (a **fellowship**). Osteopathic training additionally incorporates physical therapies devoted to the musculoskeletal system to diagnose and treat illness. The terms **physician, doctor,** and

practitioner are all ways to describe these medical professionals. A **physician assistant** is trained to diagnose, treat, and prescribe medication as part of a healthcare team (usually with a supervising physician). A **nurse practitioner** is a registered nurse who has completed nursing school and then advanced training to diagnose, treat, and prescribe medications. In many states, NPs are independent practitioners. In a few others, NPs work with a supervising physician. All of these professionals may provide primary care.

Find out if the doctor has any recent disciplinary actions (usually within the last five years), and if so, what the issue was and how the board managed the problem (probation, monitoring, re-training, etc.). Some red-flag issues in the report might include multiple disciplinary issues, sexual misconduct, substance abuse, or problems with professional understanding (**competence**).

4. Explore other websites. If you have a specific condition, great resources to find doctors are patient-organization websites that include lists of doctors who treat the condition. Doctor-rating sites on the Internet are also an option. These sites are like your favorite restaurant-rating sites, though; a person who had an exceptionally bad or good experience is likely to post a review, but the average person does not always post something. Sometimes competitors post negative reviews posing as a regular person, so the best sites verify that the reviewer is an actual patient. Clearly, if a doctor has many bad reviews, it would be wise to stay away. Otherwise, ratings are just one more thing to consider while you decide for yourself.

5. Check the doctor's website. It may be helpful to see the doctor's training and interests. For example, you may want to find a doctor that offers **integrative medicine,** which means they incorporate Western medicine as well as traditional Eastern medicine options such as acupuncture. There are primary care physicians who focus their practice on particular areas, such as **geriatrics** (care of the elderly patient), pain medicine, **obstetrics** (care of pregnancy), or sports medicine.

6. If possible, ask a patient. Find out if the office returns calls promptly, if it is difficult to get an appointment, and if there is good communication of results. A well-run office is just as important to your care as the doctor is. As a patient, I've wondered what to make of receiving my lab bill before my lab results. Even in a good office, sometimes things fall through the cracks, but you want to feel confident that most of the time, the office will not let you down.

7. Make an appointment and interview the doctor. Ultimately, your instincts are your best guide. The worksheet exercise at the end of this chapter is a checklist of things to ask and notice to get you started.

8. Once you have a primary care doctor, work with them. Do ten minutes of preparation the evening before your appointment. It's all too easy to forget the questions you'd like help with when you finally get in the room. I've forgotten to ask important questions at my own doctor's visits in all the rush. My solution is to send myself a text of questions I come up with the night before. Bring any notes or results you have from other doctors, especially from the emergency room, urgent care, or specialists. Many times, those notes will not reach your doctor for several days, which is not useful for your appointment. Take your pill bottles along and do not forget your PHR.

9. Take a picture or track your problem. As they say, a picture is worth a thousand words. In medicine, pictures of things like rashes, bruises, or swelling really help, especially if the problem has changed or gone away before you got to the doctor. Cell phone cameras are a handy way to document your problem. I had a friend whose child had crossed eyes that came and went. It was always normal when she went to the doctor, so she was advised not to worry. I suggested that she photograph her daughter's crossed eyes a few times and show the pictures to her doctor. The photographs led to corrective surgery.

If you have a problem that comes and goes like pain, diarrhea, or headaches, keeping a calendar of your symptom and details such as what you ate can shed some light on the problem. (Again, cell phone calendars are handy and there might be a phone app specifically for your problem.) For example, a woman can learn that her headaches relate to her menstrual cycle, or a man may discover that his diarrhea occurs after he eats dairy products.

10. Get to know the other players of your doctor's team. Most doctors have a nurse and/or a **medical assistant** (**MA**) who will take your vital signs and start your visit. They also answer messages and relay information between doctors and patients. This is a key person to help you with your visit goals and to offer suggestions on how to meet them. Share what you need or questions you have for the visit with them.

11. Take notes freely and ask if something does not make sense. Research suggests it is difficult to recall more than about one-third of a doctor's visit. If you receive bad news, the recall rate is even worse. If you do not understand something, ask for more information. This is the doctor's failing, not yours. I've included a second worksheet in this chapter with suggestions on ways to ask common questions. If you're not getting the answers you want back, it's likely time to find a new doctor. Taking notes will give you something to refresh your memory when you leave the office.

12. Summarize. At the end of each visit ask, "How should I summarize this visit and these tests in my PHR?" and write down the answer. Not every visit needs an entry, but important changes do.

13. Leave with an action plan. Once you've summarized the visit together, what are the to-do items for you and your doctor? The most basic question to answer is when you need to come in next. Others include setting up your medication refill schedule or your next set of lab tests. Ask for as many refills as possible. If you need regular blood testing, ask for a **standing order**. This is an order the lab keeps on file so you do not need new paperwork each time.

The underlying goal of your plan should be how to stay out of the healthcare system as much as possible. For example, if you have high blood pressure and take multiple medications, set some reasonable goals with your doctor. It could be to lower your blood pressure enough to reduce the number of blood pressure medications you take. Meet this goal and you will see your doctor less, spend less money on medications, and most importantly, avoid the complications that can accompany high blood pressure, like a stroke or a heart attack. Be as specific as possible. This example plan may look like this:

a. Lose one pound per week until next appointment.

b. Research and follow a low-salt diet called the DASH diet.

c. Exercise for thirty minutes a day, four days per week.

d. Start the nicotine patch to stop smoking within six months.

e. Measure your own blood pressure at home once every three days and keep a record.

f. Return to the office in three months to review the blood pressure record to decide if you can stop one or more blood pressure medications.

g. Reassess whether you need additional services or medications to quit smoking at the next visit.

WORKSHEET

Choose and Use Your Primary Care Doctor

Here are some helpful things to notice or ask the doctor to help determine if you are choosing and using your doctor well. Cross out those that do not apply or are not that important to you.

Office Standards

☐ Making an appointment is easy.

☐ Appointments are available within twenty-four to forty-eight hours.

☐ The office seems organized.

☐ The office staff are friendly and do not treat me like a nuisance.

☐ The office has good parking and a convenient location.

☐ The office has the early/late/weekend availability I need.

☐ I want an office with a laboratory inside.

☐ My kids and/or spouse can go to the same office.

☐ They have other types of providers as well—e.g., nurse practitioners (NP), physician assistants (PA), nutritionists, etc.

☐ I can request an appointment with my doctor directly if I do not want to see the PA or NP.

☐ The appointment was on time or the delay was explained to me (delays do happen—emergencies come up or a patient needs more time for a serious problem).

☐ My privacy was respected and I did not overhear a lot of other patients' information.

Pre-Appointment

☐ Decide whether you should bring someone with (particularly if you're expecting serious news).

☐ Bring any papers or results from tests you had done elsewhere that apply to the visit (such as emergency-room discharge papers).

☐ Bring your medication list or your pill bottles.

☐ Bring note paper to jot things down during your appointment.

☐ Write your questions down or text them to yourself.

The Doctor Visit

☐ The doctor made eye contact and was respectful.

☐ The doctor listened to me without too much interruption.

☐ The doctor's examination did not make me feel unsafe or uncomfortable.

☐ The doctor answered my questions well.

☐ I was able to leave with a clear plan of when I should come back and what to do to manage my own health.

At the End of the Appointment

☐ If necessary, request a second opinion.

☐ Summarize the visit for your personal health record.

☐ Leave with an action plan and schedule your next visit.

WORKSHEET

Some Phrases To Try in the Doctor's Office

1. **Scenario: Your doctor is using too many medical words.**

   I am finding some of these terms confusing. Can you say that again in plain English?

   Repeat the term you don't understand as a question. (e.g., Nephrogenic?)

2. **Scenario: You want a second opinion.**

   Who would you recommend I see to consider this more?

3. **Scenario: You wonder if you really need that test.**

   Do you have an idea what this test might show?

   Do you think the benefits of this test outweigh the risks for me?

   What could happen if I do not have this test?

4. **Scenario: You aren't sure whether you really should have a treatment offered.**

   What would you do if I were your mom/dad/sister/brother?

   Who would you recommend I see to consider this more?

5. **Scenario: The doctor asks you a yes/no question, but you would like to explain your circumstances first.**

   I am sorry; I cannot answer that question easily. I need to share a bit of background with you on this issue first.

6. Scenario: Your doctor seems to be ordering many tests and you don't know why.

What are these tests going to tell us?

How will the results of this test change my health?

7. Scenario: You did not understand the information.

I did not understand what you said. Can you please say this a different way for me?

I am now going to repeat back what I heard. Can you please correct me where necessary?

8. Scenario: The doctor offers you a sample of a new medication you know you cannot afford to buy when you run out of the samples. (See chapter 4 for more on medication choices.)

I am worried about whether I can afford this name-brand medicine when the samples run out. Is it my best choice or is there a generic option out there that I could try first?

I am trying to get as many of my medications from the four-dollar list of drugs as possible. Can you think of one that might work here?

Your own questions and/or your selection of questions from the Agency for Healthcare Research and Quality (see the Resource Box for this website):

_____

_____

_____

_____

_____

SPECIALTY CARE

Specialty care operates a little differently than primary care. Generally, your family doctor will select a specialist based on the problem you have and their experience with a particular specialist in that field. You can make requests, like a male or female specialist or someone located near your home. Your doctor's office will likely have a **Referral Coordinator** who will work with you to set up the appointment. If you are unsatisfied after your first appointment with the specialist, ask your primary care doctor for a new referral and tell your doctor why so that they have a chance to change their referral choice in the future.

Many specialists require that a referral come from another doctor. Some do allow you to refer yourself—a **self-referral.** The advantage of self-referral can be that you save the cost of a visit with your primary care doctor if your problem is straightforward or you do not have a primary care doctor. Or you may want to self-refer because your primary care doctor is not taking action on your symptoms. For example, you may feel depressed and your doctor disagrees and will not refer you to a specialist (in which case, you probably need a new doctor). You may then want to self-refer to a mental-health specialist, such as a psychiatrist. I have included a list of common specialties here for your reference.

When self-referring, it's important to understand that it can be difficult to select the appropriate specialty. This is because many conditions are treatable by multiple specialties, with very different treatments offered by each one. For back pain, you could see a neurologist, neurosurgeon, orthopedic surgeon, pain-management physician, or a physiatrist. Each one of these specialists will treat your pain in different ways. Your primary care doctor is helpful to steer you to the most appropriate specialist, which avoids needless appointments and potential therapies that are not right for you. For example, if you have back pain and you do not want surgery, then a neurosurgeon or orthopedic surgeon is not the right choice, because surgery is their primary means of treatment.

Another potential benefit from getting a referral from a primary care doctor is to share specific details of your health history with a specialist, such as your results from past tests and treatments. Your doctor's office will share these past results with the specialist and summarize your conditions. In contrast, if you self-refer, the specialist will likely repeat tests because the results are not available. To limit repetition, get a copy of your prior test results before you make a self-referral. Finally, ask the specialists for their notes, update your PHR, and share the notes with your primary care doctor.

WHICH "OLOGIST" FOR WHAT?

(Note: There are subspecialties within a specialty. For example, there are neurologists who subspecialize in movement disorders. This would be a good choice of doctor for someone with Parkinson's disease.)

Problem	Medical Specialists	Surgical Specialists
Skin	Dermatologist	Plastic Surgeon
Head and Neck	Internal Medicine	Otolaryngologist (ENT)
Eyes	Ophthalmologist	Ophthalmologist
Cancer	Medical Oncologist	Surgical Oncologist
Stomach/Bowel	Gastroenterologist	General Surgeon

Problem	Medical Specialists	Surgical Specialists
Kidneys	Nephrologist	Urologist
Male Organs	Urologist	Urologist
Female Organs	Gynecologists	Gynecologists
Pregnancy	Obstetrician	Obstetrician
Bones and Joints	Rheumatologist	Orthopedic Surgeon
Nerves and Brain	Neurologist	Neurosurgeon
Pain	Physiatrist (also provide rehabilitation for injuries and disabilities)	Anesthesiologist
Mental health issue	Psychiatrist	
Children	Pediatrician	
Elderly	Geriatrician	

RESOURCE BOX

Find A Primary Care Doctor With Reduced Costs

findahealthcenter.hrsa.gov—Type in your zip code and find a health center that will provide care based on your income.

Alternatives to Insurance-covered Primary Care

dpcare.org—Discusses the principles of direct primary care and helps you find a direct primary care provider in your area.

aapp.org—Provides information about concierge care and lists local concierge physicians.

Questions to Ask At Doctor Visits

ahrq.gov/patients-consumers/patient-in-volvement/ask-your-doctor—Lists questions and has useful videos and other tools to help you communicate your needs at the doctor's office.

CHAPTER 6
Participate in Test and Treatment Decisions

Winning is overrated. The only time it is
really important is in surgery and war.
Al McGuire

Normal test results can be very reassuring, but medical testing is not a perfect science. If the average healthy person has twenty laboratory tests, we statistically expect that one of them will come back abnormal. Every test has a false positive rate and a false negative rate. Because of such error, the more testing you have done, the more likely you will have an abnormal positive or negative result. An incorrect positive result is a **false positive** and an incorrect negative result is a **false negative.** A growing number of experts are concerned that we have become a testing society and that this has not led to better patient health at all.

You are probably thinking, "So why should I have to worry about this. Shouldn't I be able to go with what my doctors recommend?" The goal of this chapter is certainly not to undermine your relationship with your doctors. Rather, the goal is to engage you in the decision-making process, because it is often more complex than a yes/no decision. The goal is to test when necessary to improve your health and as a joint decision. Working together with your doctor to make your best health choice is called **shared decision-making.**

Every health decision is worthy of some consideration not only because of error rates and because all tests have risks (like bleeding, infection, and even death). In addition, ideas and habits in medicine change over time. For example, it is commonplace to order a **computed tomography scan (CT).** We are now aware that there may be long-term health effects from too many of them, particularly in children.) This is because a CT doses a significant amount of radiation to the person getting the test (like dozens of x-rays at once). Radiation, when accumulated in the body, has negative health consequences, including an increased risk of cancer. As we understand this more, ordering CTs may not be so commonplace in the future.

Here are some guiding principles to help you participate in your healthcare decisions (see the Resource Box for more in-depth guidance):

1. Start by asking what the risks, benefits, and alternatives to treatment are. Choosing tests and treatments wisely starts with being informed. **Informed consent** means you have decided to do the test or have the treatment after learning the important risks, benefits, and alternatives. The doctor should explain these to you in plain English. Be sure to clarify anything that does not make sense to you, and take your time. You do not have to decide anything at that moment. If you are still unsure, consider seeing a different doctor or doctors to explore other points of view (a **second opinion**).

2. Go back to your Internet research (chapter 2). Fancy treatments get a lot of free marketing on medical TV programming. The exciting medical breakthroughs are often expensive tests and not well covered by insurance. Sometimes they're not even breakthroughs, just existing treatments with great marketing. One such example is laser surgery. Saying laser implies impressive, modern technology, yet laser surgery is not new at all. What are new are private laser centers that manage to market the idea as a new one. Laser surgeries can cost significantly more than routine surgery, and there may not be supporting scientific evidence that laser surgery is the superior option. If offered a new therapy, research the topic to see if it really is a breakthrough and what other options you have. Finally, consider a second opinion.

3. Personalize testing recommendations. Blood tests, prostate and breast exams, mammograms, and colonoscopies are all common tests offered at different stages of life. They are **screening tests** that have been studied over time and found to make a difference in preventing a disease altogether or improving the treatment results through earlier detection. **Colonoscopies** (colon inspection via a camera) can visualize colon cancers or pre-cancers. Removal of a pre-cancerous growth can avoid colon cancer. If there is a cancer, early treatment is simpler and can reduce the likelihood of death from colon cancer.

Screening guidelines set out what type of people (gender, age, race, and medical-risk factors) should be screened and the screening interval (e.g., every year versus every five or ten years). These recommendations can change over time based on newer research. The **US Preventive Services Task Force (USPTF)** is the government agency assigned to analyze the research and then make screening recommendations. Screening recommendations can be confusing because other professional organizations often publish different screening guidelines. For example, the USPTF recommends screening mammograms in women over the age of fifty. Some medical organizations believe this age should be forty. The USPTF is currently reviewing current breast-cancer research to decide if it should change the guideline.

Ultimately, you and your doctor need to weigh the public screening recommendations against your personal risks to determine when you should start screening for a certain disease. Personal risk is determined from things like your age, current health, and your family history. A person with a strong family history of cancer, or a personal past history of smoking, has an increased personal risk of certain cancers. This person may need to begin screening earlier than the USPTF recommendation.

In the future, screening guidelines may become obsolete. Instead, we may just do a genetic test to decide if your personal risk for a disease is high enough to warrant more investigation or even start treatment. This approach is termed **personalized medicine,** and it has already begun for certain diseases and treatments.

4. Surgery is worth some extra attention. Surgery can be lifesaving and necessary. Other times, there are non-surgical (often called **conservative**) treatment options to consider. As an estimated one hundred fifty thousand Americans die each year from surgery (half of those from avoidable causes), having surgery clearly is an important decision for your participation.

A good example to help demonstrate the importance of exploring your options is back pain. Many people over fifty years of age have back pain. A CT or MRI of the back by this age is rarely perfect. There is usually some kind of abnormality, such as a bulging disk, arthritis, or a narrowing of the spinal canal (**stenosis**). Some research shows that patients with back pain who have a CT or MRI have the same cure rates for their back pain as patients who never had a CT or MRI. The people with an abnormal MRI or CT in these studies often had surgery but did not necessarily get relief from their back pain. The people who did not have a CT or MRI did not have surgery. This means that some of the people who had surgery took surgical risks but received no benefit, and they may have improved with just conservative therapy.

Conservative initial therapies include medications, injections, and physical therapy.

If conservative therapies do not work, there can be several surgical options to review. **Interventional radiologists** and **anesthesiologists**, for example, can treat some back conditions with targeted injections of medication or tiny manipulations under intermittent X-ray guidance (**fluoroscopy**). **Laparoscopic surgery**—surgery through tiny incisions and with the aid of a camera—could be an option. In addition, sometimes smaller-than-traditional incisions (**minimally invasive surgery**) are an option.

The worksheet here provides some questions to help put the shared decision-making model into practice if you are considering surgery.

RESOURCE BOX

Health Decision-making

effectivehealthcare.ahrq.gov—This website offers treatment summaries, interactive testing, and treatment decision-making tools.

choosingwisely.org—Here, a collection of professional medical groups have listed at least five areas of testing per specialty for discussion between patients and doctors.

informedmedicaldecisions.org—Learn more about the Shared Decision-making Model and access tools to learn how to participate in healthcare decisions.

curetogether.com—International site that lists the treatment options for various diseases.

participatorymedicine.org—A nonprofit organization that brings together patients and providers with research and information on how patients can navigate their own health.

labtestsonline.org—A website to find out what a lab test is for, normal values, and the strength of evidence for having the test done.

Health Screening

uspreventiveservicestaskforce.org—Up-to-date and evidence-based screening recommendations from the US Centers for Disease Control and Prevention (CDC).

fda.gov/scienceresearch/specialtopics/personalizedmedicine—Presents an overview and current research on personalized medicine.

Many large hospitals (e.g., Mayo Clinic, Cleveland Clinic) publish screening guidelines on their websites, as do many specialty organizations (e.g., American Cancer Society, American Diabetes Association, American Heart Association).

WORKSHEET

Questions to Ask Your Surgeon

☐ How is this surgery better than taking medicine?

☐ Are there any conservative therapies available for me to try?

☐ Is there a less invasive surgical option?

☐ What surgical options are available that you do not perform?

☐ How long will I be off from work after surgery?

☐ What activity restrictions will I have and for how long?

☐ May I speak to a patient who has had this procedure?

☐ What risk from this surgery gives you the most concern?

☐ What are my inpatient and outpatient surgical options?

☐ Would testing my tissues (pathology) at the time of my surgery possibly change your choice of surgical procedure?

(Find more at ahrq.gov/patients-consumers/patient-involvement/ ask-your-doctor)

_____

_____

_____

CHAPTER 7
Think About Dying

In this world nothing can be said to be certain, except death and taxes.
Benjamin Franklin

In modern healthcare, people receive a lot of treatment because we can provide it. This occurs even at the end stages of a disease, where little good is accomplished. It's sad to hear families say, "Given another chance, we would have said no to all of the treatments offered and just enjoyed his/her last moments at home." It's so hard for families to know when to say "No more." In other words, once the roller coaster of treatment begins, it can be very difficult to get off. Making your wishes clear before a health crisis is the best step to avoid an unwanted ride.

An **advanced directive** is your official written instructions for the type of care you would like (sometimes referred to as a **living will**) and whom you authorize to make medical decisions for you if you cannot speak for yourself (a **durable power of attorney for healthcare**).

Life-sustaining care is full care, and it has two aspects. If your heart or lungs stop working, treatment includes chest compressions, medications, blood products, and artificial breathing. This is **CPR (cardiopulmonary resuscitation)**. After CPR, you may continue to need artificial breathing through a tube attached to a special machine (**intubation**) along with medications as necessary to keep you alive. In the hospital, a patient's wish to not receive CPR has a **DNR** order, which stands for **do not resuscitate**. The second part of life-sustaining care is providing nutrition and hydration, even if by artificial means, like an **intravenous line** in a vein (**IV**) or a tube to your stomach.

The alternative to life-sustaining care is **comfort care**. Comfort care includes personal hygiene (e.g., bathing) and medication for pain or other physical symptoms. It includes psychosocial and spiritual support. Curing the disease is not the focus because that is the less likely outcome. This is sometimes termed **palliative care**. **Hospice** refers to palliative care provided outside of a hospital in a special facility or in your home. Delivery of hospice care occurs through a variety of people from physical, social, and spiritual disciplines.

While a cure or life-sustaining treatment is not the focus, a patient can choose to have such treatments while under hospice care. If the patient has Medicare, a healthcare professional must certify that the person is unlikely to live more than six months, even with treatment. However, an unlimited amount of sixty-day extensions are available if the diagnosis does not run its expected course. Palliative care is then fully covered. However, Medicare hospice coverage does not cover room and board costs or any medication that is not part of the palliative care.

Below are several health scenarios to help you think about when you would want life-sustaining care and when you would prefer comfort measures only. This is the starting point to creating an advanced directive.

1. What would I want if I had a condition that left me in a persistent vegetative state? People often say, "I definitely do not want to be kept alive as a vegetable." This refers to an extreme state of poor recovery, which is medically termed a **persistent vegetative state.** This means the body is only partially conscious and unable to perform many acts of free will. Generally, in order to make this diagnosis, there are several tests of a person's brain function and two or more doctors must agree that this is the correct diagnosis.

2. What kind of care would I want in an acute, serious condition where, if I survive, I would have some permanent losses? Common examples of this type of condition would be after a stroke or a bad car accident. Consider if you are paralyzed on one side, confined to a wheelchair, or unable to speak. Would your preferences differ in each of these circumstances?

3. What kind of care would I want if diagnosed with a chronic condition that was not terminal but would reduce my functioning over time? Examples of these conditions are **Parkinson's disease** or **Multiple Sclerosis**, where motor strength and ability can progressively decline. Also consider conditions that cause **dementia,** such as **Alzheimer's disease**, where your ability to think and mentally function will progressively decline.

4. What kind of care would I want if I had a terminal condition? A **terminal condition** is one that is likely to end your life, even with treatment. An example of a terminal condition is advanced cancer that has spread to other areas (**metastasized**), such as to the brain, bone, liver, or lungs.

5. Do I want to donate my organs? Eligibility to donate depends on what organs you want to donate (common ones are eyes, heart, liver, or kidneys) and the condition of the organ. If you have strong feelings about organ donation either way, you should include them in your living will. Otherwise, this question may be posed to your family to decide at a difficult time.

6. Do I want an autopsy performed on my body? Sometimes an autopsy is a legal requirement, but other times you can request one. For example, you may have a condition that you want your family to learn more about because it possibly affects them as well. An autopsy could provide some of this information.

7. Do I have specific beliefs that will affect my care? You have the right to request care in line with your beliefs. For example, blood transfusions are against the beliefs of many people of the Jehovah's Witness faith. Since blood transfusion is a life-sustaining treatment, it will be part of your emergency treatment without clear instructions from you otherwise. Some ideas are to keep instructions in your wallet, wear an ID bracelet, or find out if your state has a public registry to record your wishes, as discussed later in this chapter.

The second component to an advanced directive is to identify the person you would like to make healthcare decisions for you if you are unable to do so. This document is a **durable power of attorney (POA) for healthcare**. This person may make healthcare decisions in your place when you cannot speak for yourself. Other names for this role are **healthcare proxy** or **healthcare surrogate.** There are all kinds of POAs, such as financial or legal. While you may use the same person for multiple POAs, a healthcare POA must have a separate document altogether.

Your POA for healthcare should be a person who knows you well enough to understand and carry out your wishes; both are equally important requirements. Some people cannot bring themselves to say no to treatment for a loved one when the time comes. Others may not be able to withstand pressure from family members who may not agree with your decision. If you cannot find a suitable candidate, select an attorney or pay a professional healthcare POA.

Why both a healthcare POA and a living will? Because a living will by itself cannot handle all of the grey zones between a full recovery and a persistent vegetative state. It is simply too difficult to put all health situations into words. For example, it's not always clear whether a patient could recover with some nutrition, and a short trial of feeding could help to clarify this. Your healthcare POA would make that call on your behalf.

These are all difficult scenarios to think about, let alone discuss, but sharing your reasons behind your decisions will help your loved ones understand them. The more time you spend on this difficult subject ahead of time, the less difficulty there will be when the time actually comes to respect your wishes. A friend, religious leader, or other neutral support person could be of assistance. Some other great resources on how to begin this conversation are included in the Resource Box below.

The Resource Box contains many services (often free) to help you make your advance directive effective in your state. Each state has legal requirements on what an advanced directive needs to look like. Other options for help include community hospital social workers or hospital patient advocates who can provide assistance, particularly if you are hospitalized. Of course, lawyers (particularly those involved in estate planning) can help you as well.

These documents periodically need updating as you get older or when your health changes. Your advanced directive is of little use if no one knows it exists. Consider carrying a wallet card that states that you have an advanced directive to notify healthcare providers. In addition, most states have an Advanced Directive Registry to store an electronic copy of your advanced directive for healthcare providers to access.

Finally, chapter 8 may be helpful to read now if you are currently involved in a serious health matter. It includes information and resources for personally having or caregiving for someone with serious illness.

RESOURCE BOX

Advanced Directives and Durable Powers of Attorney

theconversationproject.org—A website of resources and a starter kit designed to help you go through end-of-life questions and wishes with your loved ones.

americanbar.org—Enter "consumer toolkit healthcare" into the website's search bar to find resources for writing an advanced directive.

agingwithdignity.org—Planning guides and personal assistance in twenty-six languages. This site has a document called "Five Wishes," which is a living will legal in forty-three states (available online or in hard copy).

cancerlegalresourcecenter.org—This is a volunteer service of lawyers and other professionals to help patients, caregivers, and others coping with cancer who have legal issues.

www.caringinfo.org—The National Hospice and Palliative Care Organization is a national consumer support program to help improve care at the end of life. They provide free advanced directives with instructions for each state.

CHAPTER 8
Care, Support, and Advocate

It is much more important to know what sort of patient has a disease than what sort of disease the patient has.
William Osler, grandfather of Western medicine

People with support have better healthcare experiences than those without. The objective of this chapter is to help ensure you never deal with a health problem alone. It further provides some information to help if you are a **caregiver** looking after an ill person.

A support network begins with your friends and family. As with all human relationships, we expect that people will react differently to illness and some will be better supporters than others. These differences can threaten relationships. For example, there is often an otherwise helpful person in a sick person's life who is surprisingly unsupportive about the illness. They can sound callous or indifferent or do a poor job if asked to help. Often, this person is uncomfortable with illness and this is a self-protective response. Other common players are those who offer help but are too scattered and disorganized in their own life to be reliable. You may have a martyr in your midst who will burden you with reports on what they have done for you. By recognizing your own cast of characters, you can best create a realistic support roster and avoid conflicts that can have a negative effect on your well-being. This chapter includes a worksheet with a list of common tasks you could assign to people in your network who want to help.

Ideally, there is one special person who you are close to who is able and willing to do more. This person can become your **healthcare advocate**. A healthcare advocate supports and promotes your rights as a patient. In other words, this person looks out for your interests during your healthcare experience. This can be the same person who is your healthcare power of attorney (discussed in chapter 7), or it can be a different person.

Professional advocacy organizations are available at a fee. They could be a good option if you do not have local support, or for caregivers and family members who may not have the time or the ability to help as much as they would like to. The paid advocate can follow your care instructions and communicate information to all of your family. Online advocate organizations tend to be great options for insurance issues and research. Smaller boutique advocates and **geriatric care management groups** are good options in cases where a person needs coordinated care and care oversight. A few specific examples are included in the following Resource Box, but there are many similar companies on the Internet.

If you cannot identify someone you know or afford a professional advocate, check to see if your insurance company provides advocates. Sometimes, this service is free. Many hospitals now have an advocacy department for help at no charge during a hospital stay.

Another source of support is the community. Community support can help you see that you are not alone, open your eyes to new treatment options, and provide clever ideas that others with the same problems have developed. Finally, observing people at various stages of your own illness can really help you shape your own health decisions and plans. Many hospitals run free support groups for various health problems. If you cannot find a good fit with a local support group, or perhaps you prefer greater privacy, try an online community (a few are included in the Resource Box).

If your illness advances, you may need to find more services to help you. There are services available to run errands and perform household tasks. **Home healthcare** agencies and nursing agencies can provide in-home care for a specified number of hours per week or day. When care duties become very detailed or round-the-clock, you may need to move out of your home and into a **skilled nursing facility** or **rehabilitative nursing home**.

It's important to appreciate that regular health insurance does not usually cover these advanced services. For example, Medicare does not pay for long-term skilled nursing care, although it may pay for a limited amount of rehabilitative care (such as for someone recovering from surgery who will ultimately return home). As discussed in chapter 10, it's best to explore long-term care insurance while you are still well. When you actually need this type of care, you are not usually in a position to start researching and it is the most expensive time to purchase long-term-care insurance.

If you are dealing with a serious illness, this may also be a good time to review chapter 7, which discusses advanced directives and other important documents to have in place.

If you are reading this as a caregiver, you may be facing many challenges with the ill person and your own needs. Caregivers often do not take care of themselves physically or emotionally. Financially, many caregivers end up living in debt in order to take care of a loved one. Self-care, however, is necessary if you expect to take care of another person effectively. Medical research strongly supports that caregivers need some time to nurture themselves in order to keep being effective and to avoid crisis and conflict. This is **respite care**. Without it, many problems can manifest—perhaps an overtired caregiver gives the wrong dose of medication, says unkind words, or inflicts physical harm on the ill person.

There are many saboteurs to respite care. When you are a caregiver, you may have people directly or indirectly setting the expectation that you should give, give, and give more. The ill person may not be able or willing to see your needs. Your job, family, or friends may still expect you to perform at your pre-caregiver level. The only answer to all of it is for you as caregiver to provide care and comfort to yourself first. The following Resource Box provides some sources to learn about self-care and find local respite-care agencies and volunteers.

RESOURCE BOX

Support

patientslikeme.com—A large, well-established forum to connect patients with similar conditions.

Communication

caringbridge.org—A free website and app platform to keep people informed and to create a support plan and sign-up schedule for chores and errands.

carepages.com—A patient website to blog about health challenges and share experiences with friends and family.

---

memorieslive.org—A nonprofit organization that helps people with terminal illnesses make movies to preserve and share words of love and wisdom.

Caregivers

caregiveraction.org—The National Family Caregivers Association is a nonprofit advocate for caregivers. They provide free advice and information for caregivers for a wide variety of conditions.
caregiverslibrary.org—Free articles, checklists, and caregiver tools.
archrespite.org—A database of volunteers in your area that will give you a break for free and respite resources in your state.
sharethecare.org—A caregiving resource website as well as a scheduler for chores and errands.

Advocacy

patientadvocate.org—Website from the Patient Advocate Foundation; links and reports, including links on financial support and transportation.
advoconnection.com—Provides information on how to select and interview a patient advocate and a list of patient advocates in your area (it does not monitor the advocates for quality).

WORKSHEET

What Do I Need and Who Best to Help Me?

Below are some general categories of help people often need when they're ill. Think about who in your family and social network would be helpful for each category. Put his/her name under the task. Add question marks by those you are not sure about and stars by those you are. Also, consider if the task would be better suited to a paid professional instead of using your support network.

☐ Meals

☐ Financial monitoring

☐ Legal documents (powers of attorney, advanced directive, etc.)

☐ Organizing and reviewing your medical bills

☐ Driving

☐ Help in your medical appointments

☐ Confidante

☐ Help with children

☐ Relaxing

☐ Laughing

☐ Taking calls and answering questions from others

☐ Talking to your doctors, clarifying your care

CHAPTER 9
Understand Hospital Care

A hospital bed is a bed with the meter running.
Groucho Marx

By this point in the book, I hope you feel that obtaining the best healthcare absolutely requires your collaboration. Ideally, the result is that you live your life and mainly stay *out* of the healthcare system. However, nearly everyone faces a time when they have no choice but to go deep into the healthcare system. No place is deeper than the hospital, which is like a complex anthill of people who are all executing their own particular functions twenty-four hours a day, seven days a week. This chapter discusses some practical ways to participate in your healthcare in this sometimes intimidating place.

1. If possible, go to the same hospital where you last went. This saves time by not having to duplicate tests and procedures and can help you get the proper diagnosis and treatment.

2. Bring your paperwork. There is no better place to bring your Personal Health Record and/or an Advanced Directive than the hospital. Both will make your treatment decisions clearer. If you do not have these ready yet, bring all of your medication bottles and any health records that you do have.

3. Optimize comfort. Hospital care, particularly if it starts in the emergency room, can be a long process. Being comfortable helps you stay engaged in your healthcare decisions by avoiding frustration. Make important arrangements beforehand (pickup for children etc.). Dress in layers and bring food and water. Just make sure you ask a nurse before you eat or drink in case it will interfere with your care. Ideally, you should take someone along who can help you.

4. Be prepared to see people come and go. The hospital works in compartments of people, and those compartments work in shifts. If you go to the emergency room, people you may never see again will talk to and treat you. If you are sick enough to stay in the hospital (an **admission**), a completely new team will be responsible for your care. This team could then consult specialists. Feel free to ask each person who they are and why they are seeing you. Otherwise, it is easy to become frustrated with so many visits.

5. Figure out your team players. If you are admitted (are an **inpatient**), your first mission is to know who will oversee your care—your **attending physician**. This is who you need to speak with to make healthcare decisions and learn about your status. Often, this is not your own primary care physician. **Hospitalists** are doctors who work exclusively as attending physicians in the hospital. You may see a physician assistant or a nurse practitioner, who works with the attending physician (see chapter 5 for more information about the different types of treating healthcare professionals).

If you are at an **academic medical center** (hospitals associated with colleges or universities), you may see several doctors in training. The list includes **medical students** (earning a medical degree), **residents** (have a medical degree and are now getting training in their specialty), **fellows** (have a residency training and are now getting more detailed subspecialty training), and the attending physician (the one in charge of them all). Treating you is an essential part of training the new legion of doctors that will replace the attending physician one day. If the thought of doctors in training makes you overly uncomfortable, it may be best to select a hospital that is not an academic medical center.

In general, your primary team comes to visit you on **rounds** in the early morning. This is not a very convenient time for patients or families to ask questions. Ideally, you should plan your questions the evening before, or you will risk waiting another day to ask your questions. If your question is particularly urgent, ask your nurse to communicate the question during the day. Sometimes, the nurses can facilitate a telephone conference or meeting with the doctor. Since you are ill, this is particularly useful time for a healthcare advocate to help you ask questions and write down important information about your treatment and tests (review chapter 8 for more on healthcare advocates).

6. Nursing. Nurses primarily deliver your care round the clock. They generally work in eight- or twelve-hour shifts and care for a number of patients over their shift, often in different rooms. They may need to wake you up in the middle of the night to check your status, which can be difficult to get used to. **Shift change** is the meeting between the departing nurses and the replacement group to discuss the important health information and plans for the inpatients. They can only attend to urgent needs until that meeting is over. Ask what time the shift change is and try to make requests well before (like pain medication or bathroom assistance).

7. Move and Breathe. There is a whole host of complications that you are at risk for by just being in a hospital. One serious complication is **deep vein thrombosis (DVT**s), which are blood clots in your legs. These clots can break off, move into your lungs, and be life threatening. Simply moving (at the level set by your medical team) will help reduce stagnant blood in your veins that forms clots. Even if you are on bed rest, clench your leg muscles and move your legs around in bed.

Pneumonia is an infection in the lung and **atelectasis** is a collapse of parts of the lung. Shorter, shallow breaths increase the likelihood of these complications when you are in the hospital. Pain, position, and bed rest are just some of the reasons you would breathe this way. Both lung conditions cause fevers and will lengthen your hospital stay. Coughing and deep breathing keep your lungs open and clear.

8. Keep your pain well controlled. Staying comfortable decreases stress and aids in healing, breathing, and mobility. Treat your pain. Your goal is to focus on recovering quickly and getting off all pain medications as soon as possible. Sometimes you have to ask for pain medication. Do not wait until you are in extreme pain to ask. Rather, ask when the pain is mild and tolerable so you can wait if necessary. In acute pain situations, an **anesthesiologist** (a pain specialist) will set up a pump that allows you to self-medicate when you have pain. These machines have safeguards so that it will not deliver medication doses too close together and harm you. If your pain is uncontrolled with the pump settings, tell your nurse who will arrange to have the pump settings improved. Finally, if you have ever had a pain medication addiction or dependence, you need to let your team know this so they can choose your pain medications appropriately.

9. Double-check things at discharge. It is natural to want to run out of the hospital, but taking the time to understand your discharge plan before leaving will help keep you from having to come back (**readmission**). Sometimes readmission is unavoidable because you have a new problem. Unless your experience was horrific, try to return to the same hospital. They have all of your notes and the doctors are familiar with your condition. This is the ideal setting for re-treatment to avoid delays and errors in your treatment.

Leave the hospital armed with a written summary of your admission and all necessary prescriptions (including a refill of any regular medications you take). This is the important information to share with your primary care doctor and use to update your Personal Health Record. Confirm that your attending physician knows your doctor's name and mailing address. If you do not have a primary care doctor, ask to have a copy of the discharge summary sent to your home address. You may be advised to make follow-up appointments with specialists you saw in the hospital. Try to keep these appointments and ask the doctors for their discharge summary. That way, you can update your PHR without hospital records.

10. On your way home, fill your prescriptions and make a follow-up appointment with your primary care doctor. There's a lot of research that shows that completing these two simple steps within the first twenty-four hours dramatically reduces your chances of readmission to the hospital. Explain to your primary care doctor's office staff that this is a discharge appointment and must be within the week. Remember to bring your medications and all notes from your hospital stay because sometimes the hospital records do not arrive before your appointment. Even if you do not have a primary care doctor, follow-up at an urgent care center or no/low-cost clinic to ensure you are on the right track.

RESOURCE BOX

Hospital Care

medicare.gov/hospitalcompare—Search hospitals close to you by zip code and learn about each hospital's services and measurements for quality of care.

whynotthebest.org—nonprofit organization that collects different quality measures for hospitals. Review hospitals in your area or one specific hospital for measurements of the quality of care.

CHAPTER 10
Stretch Your Healthcare Dollar

*Healing is a matter of time, but it is sometimes
also a matter of opportunity.*
Hippocrates

Large medical bills are the number-one reason people declare bankruptcy in the United States. Even people who do all the right things—eat right, exercise, and reduce stress—can be the victim of an accident or cancer. Bottom line, living without health insurance is a gamble.

Insurance is the most complicated part of the healthcare system, and it's very hard to make interesting. (I was scared to put it in the middle of the book for fear you would stop reading.) This chapter helps you choose a healthcare insurance plan and use it to its greatest effect. It also includes ways to get healthcare for no or low-cost if you just cannot afford insurance at this time.

To begin, you must speak a little of the language of health insurance. The cost of your insurance plan is the **premium**. A **copayment** (often shortened to **copay**) is the fee you pay the doctor or for other medical care upfront. Your insurance company, based on your plan selection, sets the copay amounts. Cheaper plans generally have higher copays. One reason insurance companies offer copays is to motivate you to only go to the doctor when necessary and to choose cheaper care options. For example, emergency-room copays are more expensive than urgent-care copays, and office-visit copays are lower than urgent-care copays. This is because emergency-room visits cost the most to the health plans and office visits the least, with urgent care somewhere in the middle. Similarly, care that occurs without an overnight stay (**outpatient care**) is less expensive and has smaller copays than services that require an overnight stay (**inpatient care**).

Your **deductible** is the amount you pay out-of-pocket before your insurance will pay for all of your insurance bills. If your monthly premium is very high, your deductible is usually quite low, and vice-versa. There is both a **family deductible** and an **individual deductible** to meet before the insurance company will be responsible for your medical bills. For example, when a woman has a baby, the mother's care may reach her individual deductible through the costs of pregnancy and having the baby. These costs also count toward the family deductible. The baby starts at a zero credit toward his or her individual deductible and now (usually) increases the family deductible. Keep in mind that not all of the healthcare expenses you pay for count toward your deductible. Copayments often do not, as well as some types of health services (e.g., some adult vaccinations). To complicate matters more, some plans still charge a **co-insurance** fee (e.g., 20 percent of the bills after you meet your full out-of-pocket deductible).

Payments toward your deductible accumulate over a **benefit year**, which means that it resets back to zero when a new year begins. The benefit year may not be a calendar year. For example, your benefit year may begin and end in July. It's important to know when your benefit year begins and ends, particularly if you are close to reaching your full deductible amount. The end of the benefit year is a good time to schedule procedures or tests that you need but could wait to do (**elective** tests and procedures). Examples include an MRI, a colonoscopy, or surgery. If you've met your deductible for the year, you will then have fewer out-of-pocket expenses. If you wait to schedule procedures until the next benefit year, your deductible again starts at zero and you will pay all of the procedure costs until you meet the full deductible amount.

If your deductible is $5,000 and you have paid out $4,500 over the benefit year, then you will only be responsible for the next $500 of costs. For example, if you decide to schedule a $3,000 surgery, then the insurance company will cover $2,500. If you wait until your new benefit year starts, you will have to pay all of the $3,000 because your deductible has reset back to zero and you are responsible for the first $5,000 of medical charges. Meeting your deductible does not mean that all your healthcare becomes free, so call your insurance company and talk through your deductible before you make any decisions and well before the benefit year ends.

The **enrollment period** is the window of time when you can sign up for an insurance plan. This is an opportunity to ask questions about which plan is best for you. Your best plan may not be the cheapest monthly premium option. The worksheet at the end of this chapter has questions to help you select a health insurance plan. Enrollment periods are important not to miss. For example, the federal health insurance marketplace, created under the Affordable Care Act (discussed further in this chapter), has limited enrollment periods during the year, which means (aside from a few exceptions) you will need to wait until the next enrollment period to apply.

Enough with the insurance lingo. Read on to explore basics on private insurance, government insurance, and how to get no or low-cost medical attention if you are having trouble affording healthcare. The Resource Box has websites with more detail on these options.

A final general note: Always save healthcare receipts because you may be able to deduct some of your expenses on your tax return. (Check with a tax professional.)

Private Insurance

Insurance brokers are the most common private-insurance sellers. If your insurance is through your employer, your employer has already selected a broker. A broker receives a commission based on a schedule related to, among other things, the number of policies sold. If you need to purchase health insurance yourself, contact a broker or speak directly to local insurance companies to discuss available insurance options. The more complicated your health, the more you should seek out a broker who only deals with healthcare, not someone who sells insurance for healthcare, cars, houses, etc.

Insurance is expensive because it shares the health costs of all of the people in the insurance plan. Generally, older people are likely to use more healthcare. Younger people without preexisting conditions will likely use less. The plan premium charged averages out the risks among everyone.

There are more than thirty million Americans without health insurance in 2015. The Affordable Care Act is trying to reduce this number by requiring more employers to insure employees, offering government health insurance exchanges for lower-cost plans, and allowing families to insure their single children up to age twenty-six. In addition, it prohibits health insurance companies from denying coverage to someone because they have a pre-existing condition. A **pre-existing condition** is an insurance term for any health condition you have prior to your enrollment with a particular company or plan.

Even pregnancy can be a pre-existing condition. The Affordable Care Act moreover mandates that insurance companies spend less money on administrative costs and more money from premiums to promote better health for the insured people. As this law just took effect in 2014, it will take time to improve the healthcare insurance system.

There are generally two classes of plans. The first are plans with a higher monthly premium but lower out-of-pocket expenses, such as copayments and deductibles. This is a good option if you require a lot of healthcare visits, testing, and treatment.

Your second option is a **high-deductible insurance plan**, which means you initially pay out-of-pocket for healthcare services but allows you to pay them from a **Health Savings Account (HSA)**. This is a bank account only for medical expense payments. HSA banks are not traditional banks; rather, they are online. Sometimes your employer or broker selects the bank for you.

Under federal law, there is a set maximum deposit amount each year. Any money not spent can stay in the HSA account and be used the next benefit year. During that time, you may invest the money, like a 401K retirement account. Most accounts allow you to pay your bills online, and this is a handy way to organize and track your medical expenses. Many employers will match your contribution to the account. This is a great opportunity for free money. In addition, your taxable income is reduced by the amount you put into the HSA (i.e., you get to use "pre-tax dollars"), which may reduce the taxes you owe that year.

Plans with high deductibles hold the greatest benefit to people and families who are healthy because they have very few medical bills but still get the security of insurance for a large medical crisis, like a car accident or a serious diagnosis.

Once you have selected what type of private insurance is best for you, here are some ideas on how to get the most value from your purchase:

1. Find out what is included in your plan. Most insurance companies offer a number of free services that very few people use. For example, many health plans have a twenty-four-hour nurse hotline to call and ask health questions. They often offer medication cost-lowering resources and free counseling services for things like weight loss and quitting smoking. Look through your insurance plan's website or call the company to see what is included in your premium besides healthcare visits.

2. Price compare. By law, insurance companies cannot tell you where to go to get your medical treatment, but they do incentivize choices that cost them less. For example, they limit what percentage they will pay for your service. This means you will have to pay the difference if you choose an expensive place. For example, the MRI office down the street from you may be convenient to go to, but they charge nine hundred dollars. Your insurance company may only pay three hundred dollars for an MRI and can give you locations that will charge this amount. By finding this out in advance, you could save six hundred dollars of your hard-earned money. If you do not know where to start, call your insurance hotline and they can give you the closest options to you. Then call the facility to confirm the price. The Resource Box for this chapter lists websites to research average costs for procedures and tests.

3. Choose in-network healthcare practitioners when possible. An **in-network provider** has signed a contract with the insurance company to accept the set pricing of the insurance company for medical services. An **out-of-network provider** has not signed such a contract, which means there's a risk you will have to pay the doctor the difference between what your insurance company pays and the doctor's full bill. This is **balance billing**. Sometimes, your relationship with a provider will be worth the extra costs of balance billing.

Another important time to understand network relations is if you need hospital care. Sometimes, emergency-room physicians and **anes-thesiologists** (pain specialists and the ones who put you to sleep during surgery) are not in-network and will balance-bill you. Call your insurance hotline and ask which hospitals, emergency-room doctors, and anesthesiologists are in-network. (Of course this presumes you are not in an emergency at the time!) This can help determine which hospitals you should select in the future if you need healthcare.

4. Keep track of your bills and ask questions. When you receive a medical service, the provider submits a bill directly to your health insurance company. The provider generally charges one amount and the insurance plan will reduce it to a smaller amount that it has pre-set for the service. Do not pay a bill before you have received the insurance notice with the reduced amount. This statement is an **Explanation of Benefits (EOB)**.

Once you receive an EOB, compare it to the provider's bill and make sure the amounts match up. If they do not, contact the provider (the billing office number is written on the statement) to discuss the discrepancy.

If the billing issue seems more complicated or there is a lot of money at stake, ask for a payment plan and/or discuss whether it's possible to reduce the bill amount. Start with 60 to 75 percent of the total bill to allow for negotiation room. Negotiation is a particularly good option for hospital-care bills because hospitals are most familiar with writing off medical debt. There are companies that will help dispute bills and charge you based on how much they reduce your bill (see the Resource Box or search the Internet for "medical billing advocate").

5. Be cautious about changing jobs or health insurance companies. I know many people, particularly those between ages sixty and sixty-five (Medicare age), who keep working so they will have health insurance. They do not love their work, but they cannot afford to be uninsured either. Though not ideal, sometimes it makes sense to stay in a job in order to keep your health benefits.

Under the Affordable Healthcare Act, insurance companies may not deny insurance coverage based on a pre-existing condition. While this is a tremendous advance to healthcare justice, it is a new law and how effective it will be is unknown. Sometimes insurance plans have an initial **waiting period** that delay when you can get treatment for your pre-existing condition. There are also always exceptions to the rule and other ways for the insurance company to deny you coverage, so it seems wise to find out what your insurance options are and whether there will be any kind of gap in your coverage.

If you leave or lose your job, there is the potential to keep your insurance plan active under **Consolidated Omnibus Budget Reconciliation Act** legislation (**COBRA**). This federal law allows you to keep your existing employee insurance for a period of eighteen months after you leave the job. You will receive information on this option and its costs when your job ends. COBRA coverage can be expensive because you now are responsible for your premium as well as the employer portion of your premium. Many people cannot afford both portions. The bottom line is that is best to find out about the details of your COBRA plan costs before you decide to leave your job.

WORKSHEET

Choosing a Private Insurance Plan

All insurance companies have to give you a summary plan description. Start here to answer these questions, and then talk to your broker or insurance company.

1. HSA option

□ Family deductible _____

□ Individual deductible _____

□ Co-insurance _____

□ Maximum out-of-pocket expenses_____

□ Waiting period_____

□ Excluded conditions_____

2. Traditional coverage (no high deductible/HSA)

□ Deductible _____

□ Emergency room/urgent care copay_____

□ Office visit copay_____

□ Care exclusions (e.g., preventative care)?_____

□ Waiting period_____

□ Excluded conditions_____

3. For all plans, what is the prescription coverage like?

□ Medication copay_____

□ Are the prescription drugs you currently take covered by the plan? _____

4. For all plans, look at the in-network hospitals, laboratories, X-ray facilities, and doctors, and note if there are enough choices that make sense with where you live and work.

5. For all plans, run through cost scenarios with your broker or insurance company:

☐ Catastrophic illness in family (e.g., a $100,000 bill)_____

☐ No one gets sick_____

☐ If applicable, having a baby_____

6. If you have a prior condition

☐ What were last year's expenses?_____

☐ How much did you pay out-of-pocket?_____

☐ Ask if a different plan is available to result in lower out-of-pocket costs.

Government Insurance

It never hurts to look into government health programs you may qualify for to make healthcare insurance more affordable.

Medicaid is state-run health insurance for those who meet low-income and certain other requirements (e.g.,the disabled, elderly, and minors). To qualify for Medicaid, you must prove that your assets (generally not including your house or your car) and income are less than a level set by the state. Even if you have assets or income that exceeds the state minimum, you still may qualify for coverage for your children. Many children (an estimated four million or so) who would qualify are not enrolled in Medicaid. If your children get Medicaid coverage, you may then be able to afford to pay for private coverage of the adults in your household.

Medicare is a federally run health insurance program for Americans over age sixty-five, as well as those with certain disabilities and individuals with end-stage kidney disease. The insured person pays a premium for different types of coverage. The Medicare enrollment periods are only at certain times of the year. Consequently, it is best to look at the requirements the year before your sixty-fifth birthday. Medicare is a behemoth organization, and it may take a while to find the right person to talk to. An insurance broker can also be helpful. See the Resource Box in this chapter for some good Medicare resources.

Medicare **Part A** coverage is for hospital services. Physician and other health provider services are included in **Part B** coverage. **Part C** (sometimes called **Medicare Advantage)** is a program where A, B, and D benefits are provided by a private insurer and premiums are paid by Medicare. Medicare Part C is not available everywhere. Drug-coverage programs, **Part D**, are optional. Many people do not opt for Part D coverage because they have heard of something called "the gap" in that coverage where people have to pay for most of their medication expenses anyway (in 2014 it was between $2,250 and $5,100). However, even with the gap, Part D still reduces drug copays by more than 75 percent and can reduce your total deductible.

In addition, many elderly people will qualify for Medicaid, which automatically includes Part D coverage. All they have to do is enroll in Medicaid, but many people are unaware of this opportunity.

A common misconception is that once you have Medicare, all of your care is completely free. In reality, you still have some financial obligations, such as some parts of a hospital visit and some medication costs.

For example, if you are admitted to a hospital for a minimum of three days, Medicare will fully cover a certain number of days to recover in a **skilled nursing facility** (**SNF**). In 2014, only the first twenty days were fully covered, followed by a copay for days twenty-one to one hundred ($152 in 2014). After that period, you must pay all of your expenses unless you are eligible for Medicaid. (You may have to get rid of many assets to qualify).

Another useful form of care not fully covered by Medicare is **home healthcare.** This includes services provided in your home by a variety of people, such as nurses, physical therapists, and occupational therapists.

Long-term-care costs are mostly your responsibility. Besides using your savings, you can buy long-term-care insurance. The younger and healthier you are when you start your policy, the lower the monthly premium, and it's best to think about while you are well. When you actually need this type of care, you are not in an ideal position to explore your options.

Ways To Get Healthcare At Low or No Cost

There are lower- or no-cost options for care, but they can be hard to find. Here are some tips on researching your local options.

1. Start with hospitals and churches. Most county-run hospitals and churches can direct you to a free or low-cost clinic in your area. In addition, nearly every hospital (not just county hospitals) has a **compassionate care program** to treat people who need extensive care, such as essential surgery or cancer therapy, at low or no cost. You'll need to contact the hospital directly to apply.

2. Low-cost clinics—These are places to get routine care, medication refills, and lab work. You may be able to see specialists and obtain low-cost X-rays. When you're at one of these facilities, be sure to ask about other clinics and services in your area that are discounted or free, such as mammograms, dental care, and prenatal care.

3. Cash discounts—Some doctors and testing facilities will charge less if you pay cash at the time of the visit or service, as opposed to what they bill insurance for the same service. They discount the service because there are no administrative costs like billing, phone calls to the health insurance company, postage, and so on. Ask about this option when you schedule the appointment or when you check in.

4. Online care—Virtual medicine (sometimes called **telemedicine**) occurs via a webcam. It cannot treat everything, but it can be a good option for simple problems, medication refills, a time when you want additional privacy, or when you are traveling. You pay up front for your visit so you know your costs (usually less than sixty dollars).

5. Medical tourism—Identical care in other countries can be less expensive, even with travel costs. There are many medical tourism companies to help coordinate your trip. However, there is not a lot of objective information available about medical tourism risks and benefits. Research both the healthcare and cultural aspects of the country if you have an interest in medical tourism.

6. Clinical research trials—There are always studies to test available medications and treatments. If you choose to participate, all of your medications and monitoring (e.g., examinations, lab tests) will be free. Sometimes they pay cash as well. Some clinical trials are for drugs already on the market that wish to expand what conditions they can treat. Other times, a clinical trial is for a new therapy, which may be of particular interest if you have a disease that is difficult or expensive to treat. Participation in research has its risks, and you should learn about those before you decide if the study is right for you. Most studies have a **Research Coordinator** who can help you become informed. Some ways to find clinical trials are in the Resource Box.

7. Avoid the emergency department except for true emergencies. No one should hesitate to go to the emergency department because they cannot pay. The **Emergency Medical Treatment and Active Labor Act (EMTALA)** is a federal law that forbids emergency rooms (**ERs**) from turning away a person who presents to the emergency department based on ability to pay, citizenship, or legal status.

EMTALA law means emergencies and women in labor cannot be turned away. It does not mean that the ER has to cure your problem completely, however. For example, if you are having very bad pain from gallstones, the ER must treat your pain. However, they do not have to remove your gallbladder, which is the source of the pain, so you will continue to have the pain. To avoid repeat trips and more bills from the ER, you may need gallbladder surgery. If you cannot afford a larger procedure like this, explore the low-cost options discussed earlier.

Understanding that the ER is for emergencies only is very important, with or without insurance. At any hour, ER care will cost much more (at least double, but usually much more than that) than the same treatment elsewhere. Try not to wait until the evening, when every problem feels about one hundred times worse and all medical offices and urgent cares are closed.

On a final note, insurance options are always changing. If you are uninsured or have poor insurance coverage, keep going back to the insurance options described earlier in this chapter. You might find that an affordable solution has appeared or that there is a new government program just perfect for you.

RESOURCE BOX

Insurance and Cost Lowering

http://findahealthcenter.hrsa.gov/Search_ HCC.aspx—Type in your zip code and find a health center that will provide care based on your income.

naic.org—The National Association of Insurance Commissioners website. Select "Consumer Resources" and click on the option to select your state insurance department for health and other benefit programs.

healthcarebluebook.com—Research fair prices for common procedures and tests for you to compare with your own charges.

aarp.org/health—Information from the American Association of Retired Persons about medical billing and other health issues.

patientadvocate.org—The Patient Advocate Foundation explains medical bills and provides help with figuring out payment options.

www.healthcare.gov—Explore and purchase insurance options within the government marketplace.

medicare.gov—Information about what Medicare is and how to apply.

medicaid.gov—Find out whether you qualify for Medicaid, information about benefits, and how to apply.

benefits.gov—A searchable government website where you can find out what government benefits you qualify for and how to apply.

benefitscheckup.org—A government website for senior benefits including explanations about Medicare benefits.

longtermcare.gov—Explore the details and costs of long-term insurance and age-based payment options.

cdc.gov/Features/MedicalTourism—Guidance on Medical Tourism from the Center for Disease Control.

Clinical Trials

clinicaltrials.gov—A searchable database of public and private clinical research trials.

cancer.gov/clinicaltrials/—Find cancer trials sponsored by the National Cancer Institute (a government organization).

THE END

Whatever games are played with us,
we must play no games with ourselves.
Ralph Waldo Emerson

ACKNOWLEDGEMENTS

Thank you to Dr. Padma Mahant, Tara Fisher, Jesse Sanai, Brad Tritle, and Jessica Barranco for their feedback and encouragement. I am forever grateful to my husband, my mother, and the patients I have had the privilege to work with and to learn from.

ABOUT THE AUTHOR

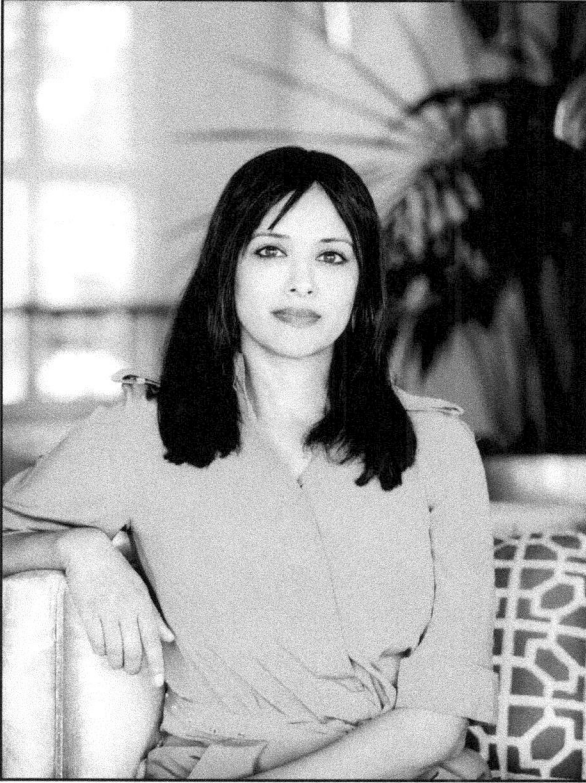

Preethy Kaibara is a family physician and healthcare attorney who likes to dream about fair, understandable healthcare and good food. She is married with three daughters and lives in Phoenix, Arizona. This is her first book.